FIREFIGHTER COLORING BOOK

FOR KIDS AGES 4 TO 6

RUBY SLIPPERS PUBLISHING

This Coloring Book Belongs To:

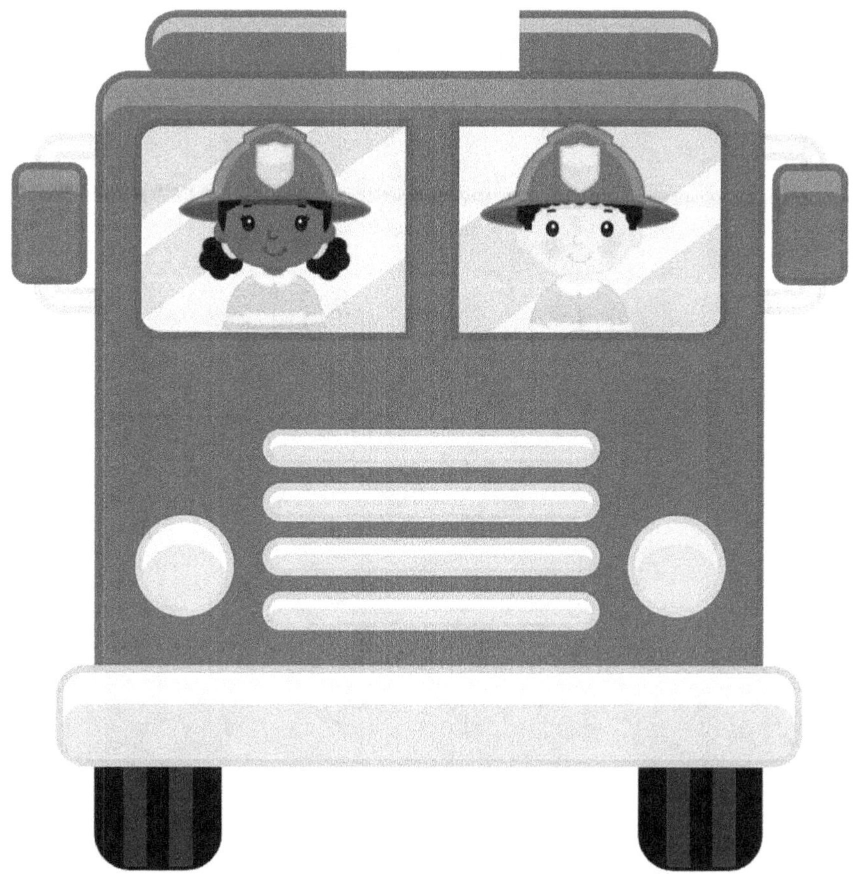

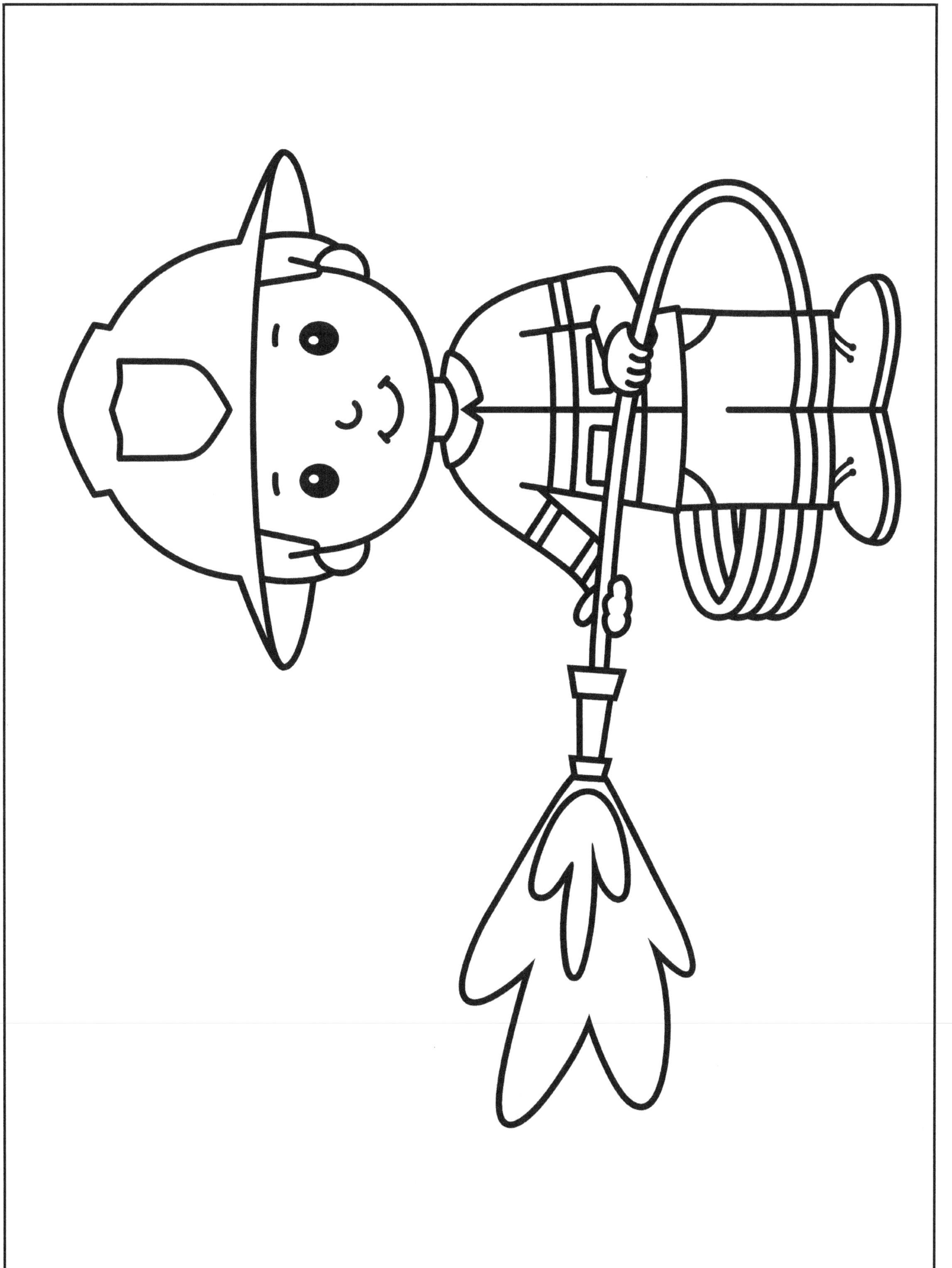

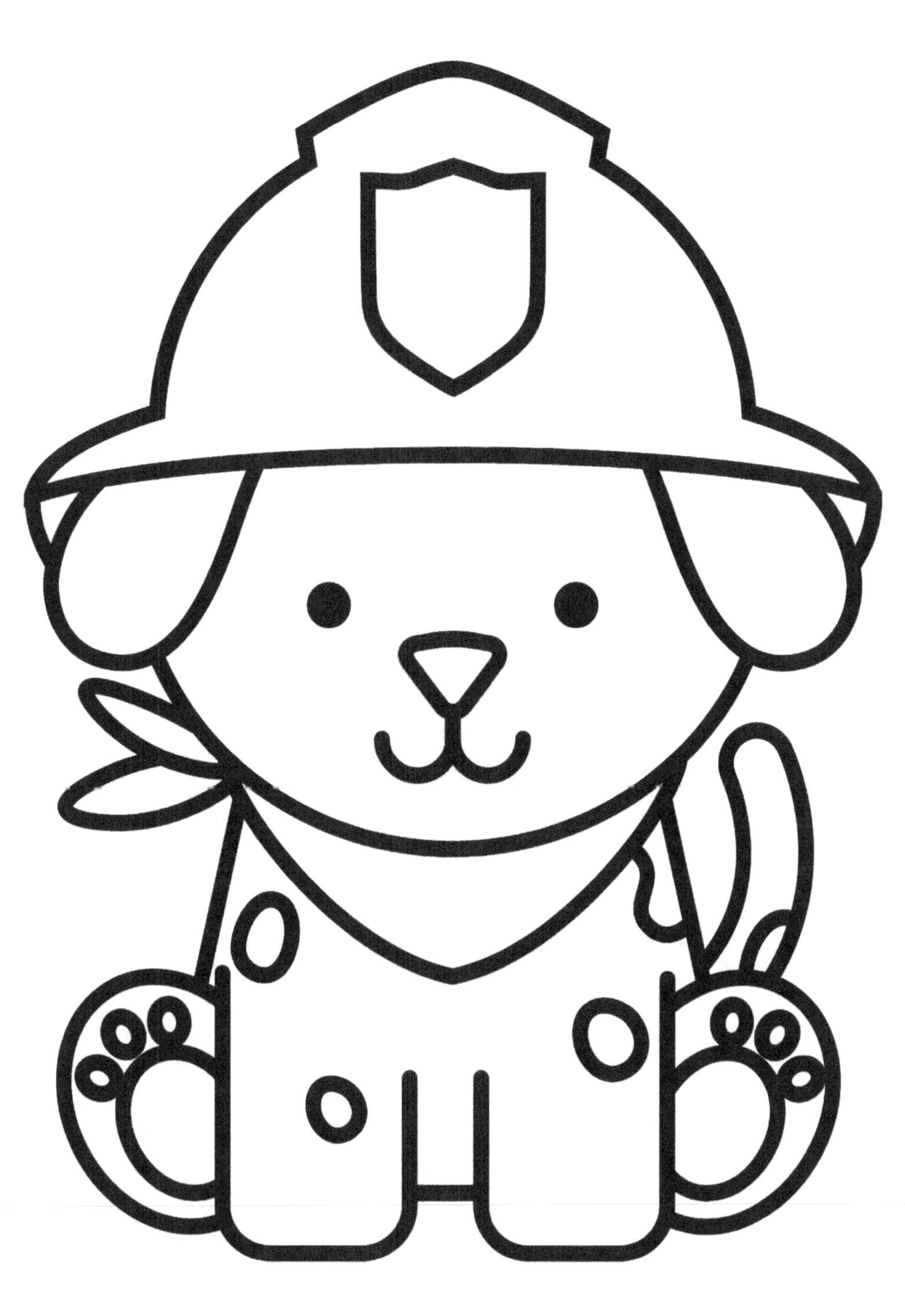

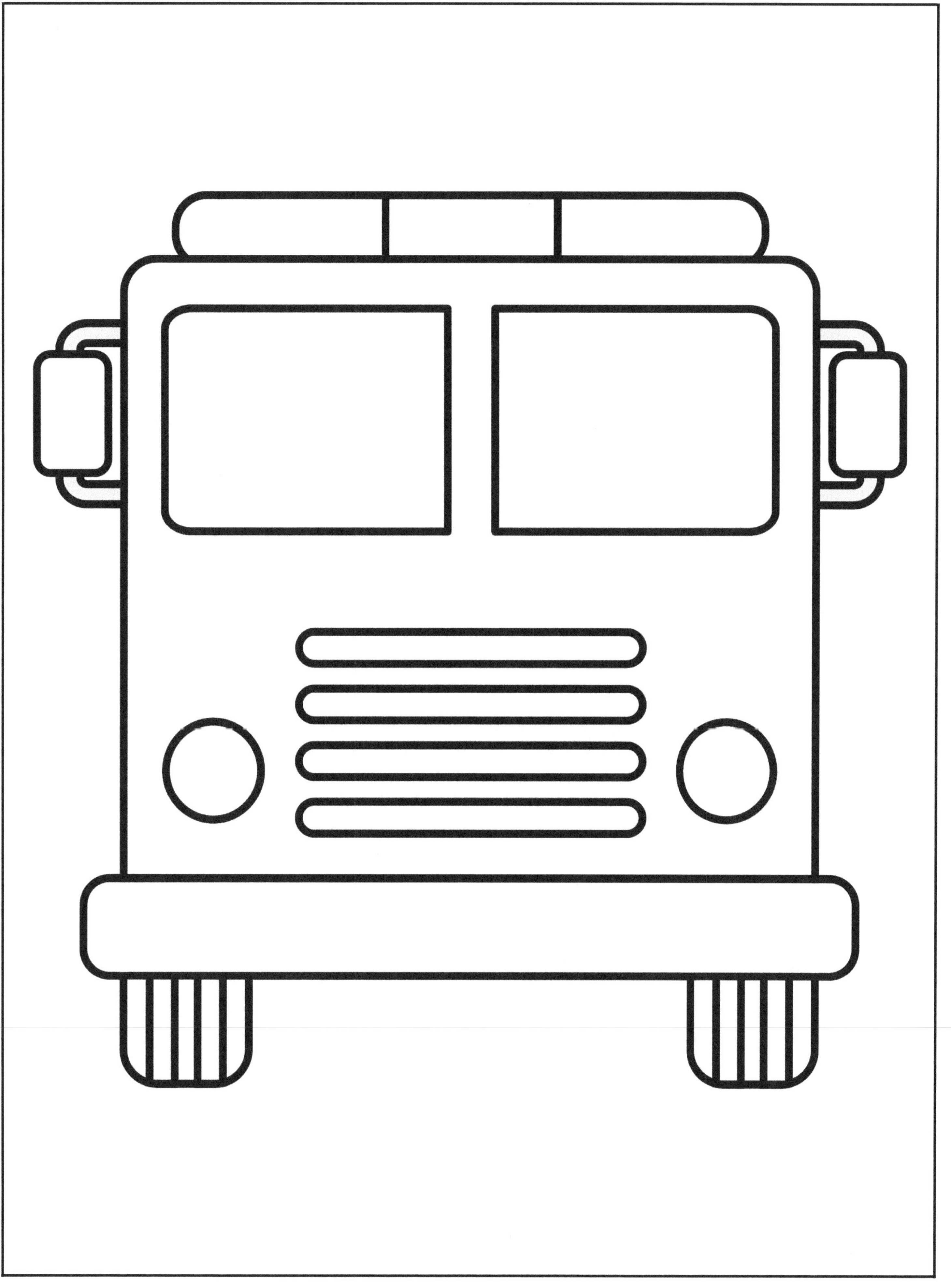

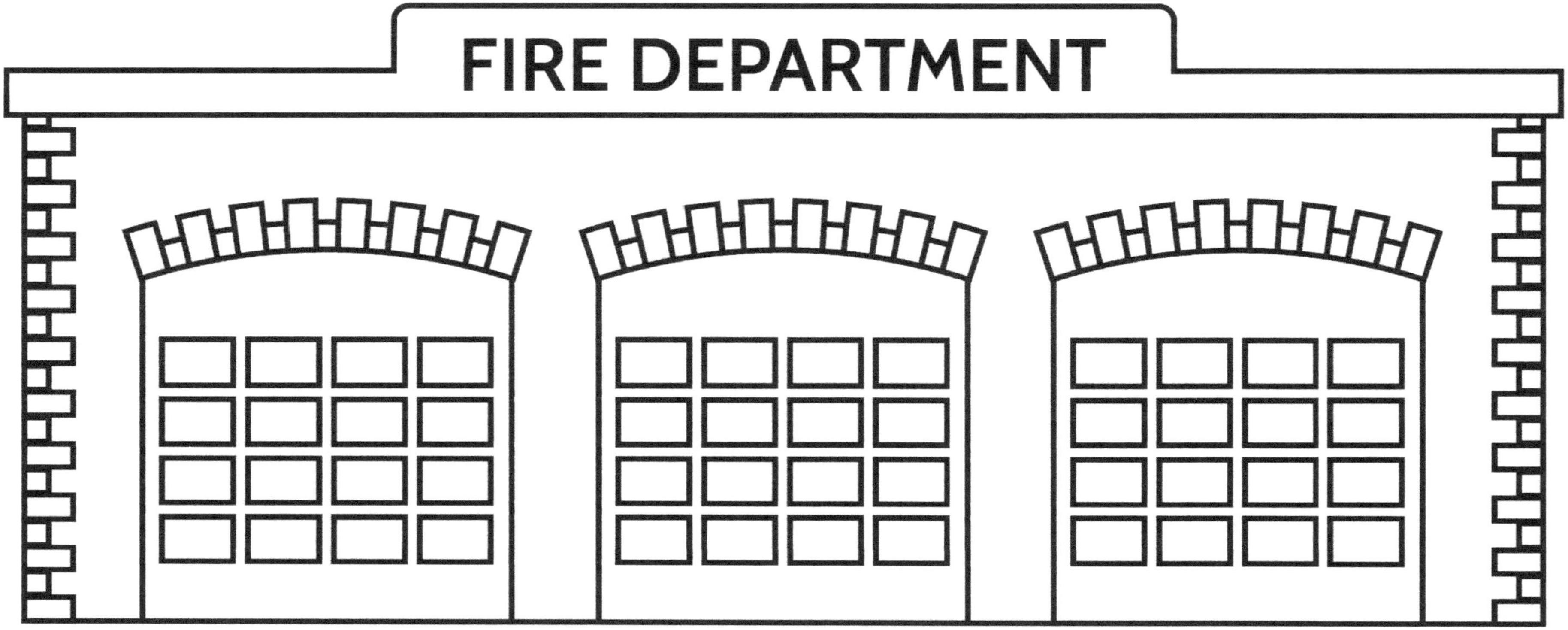

FIRE DEPARTMENT

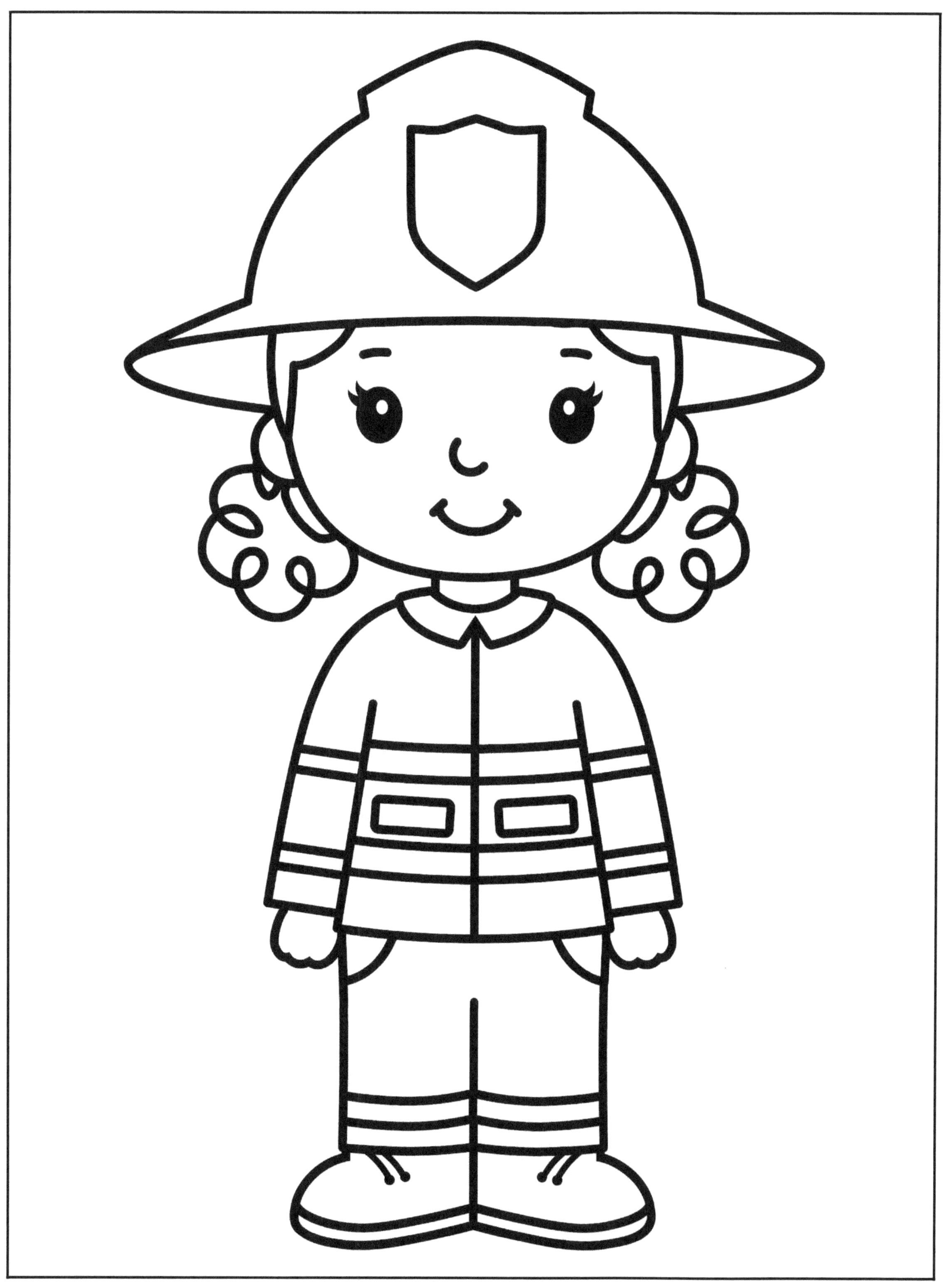

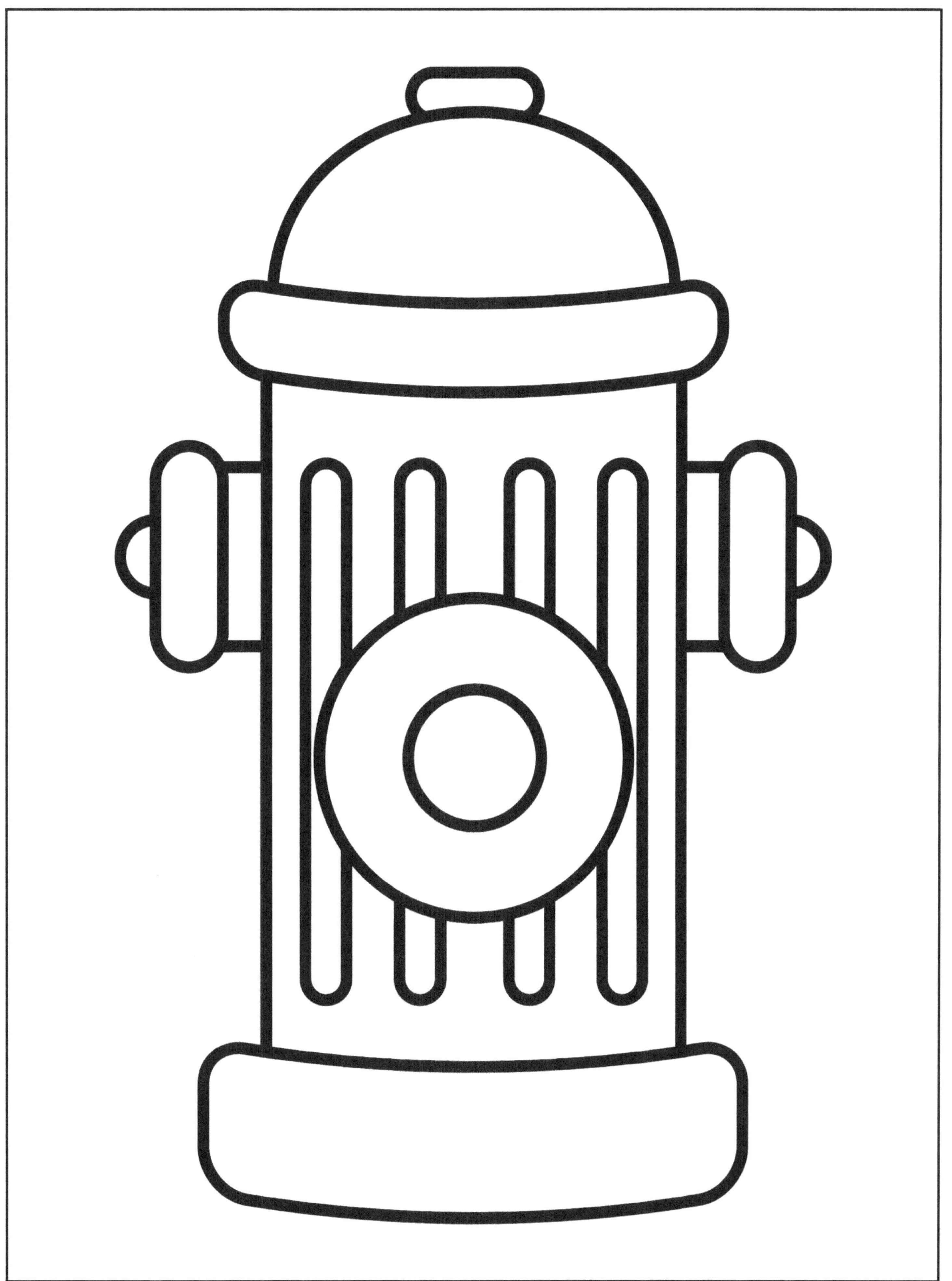

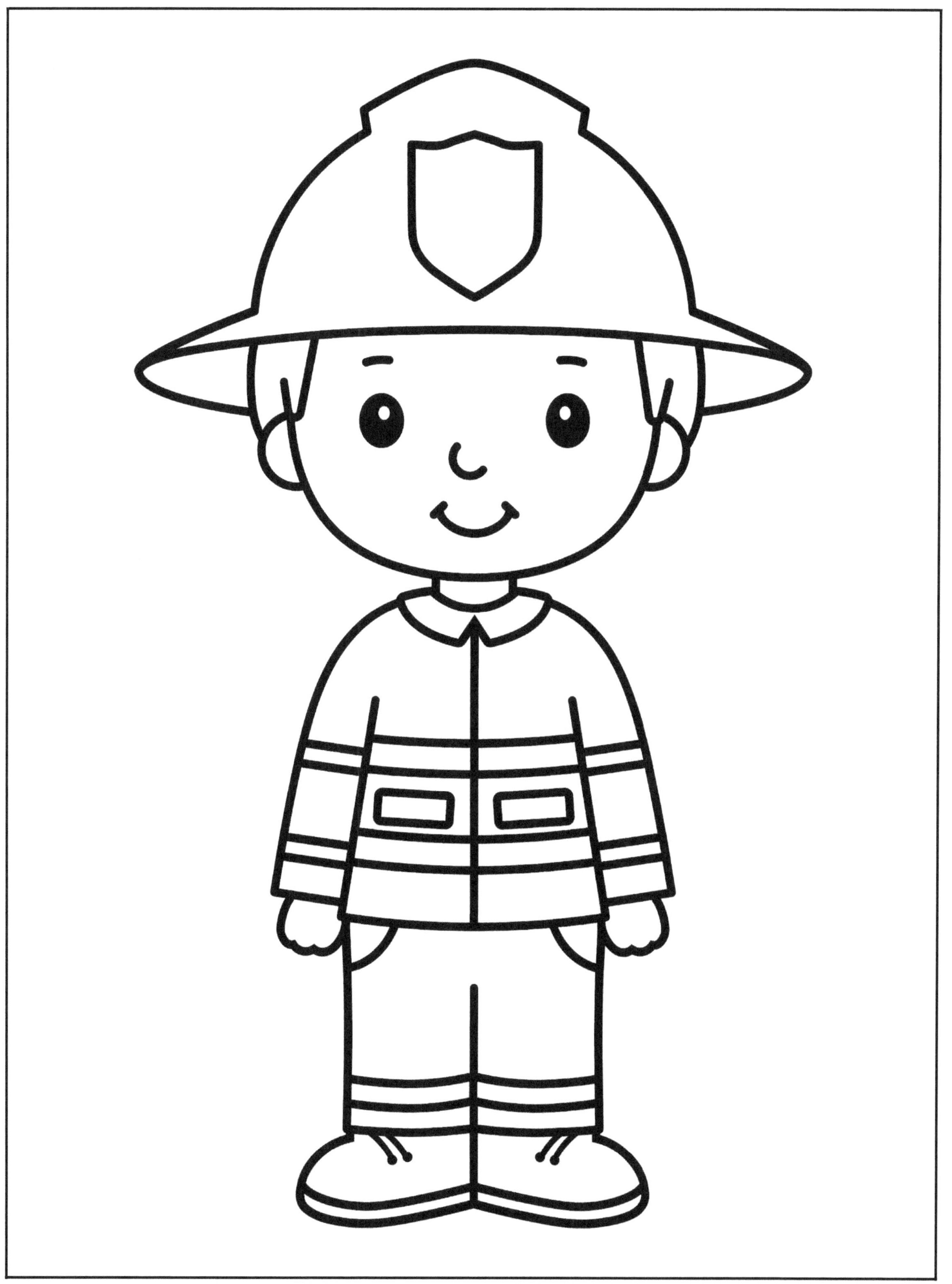

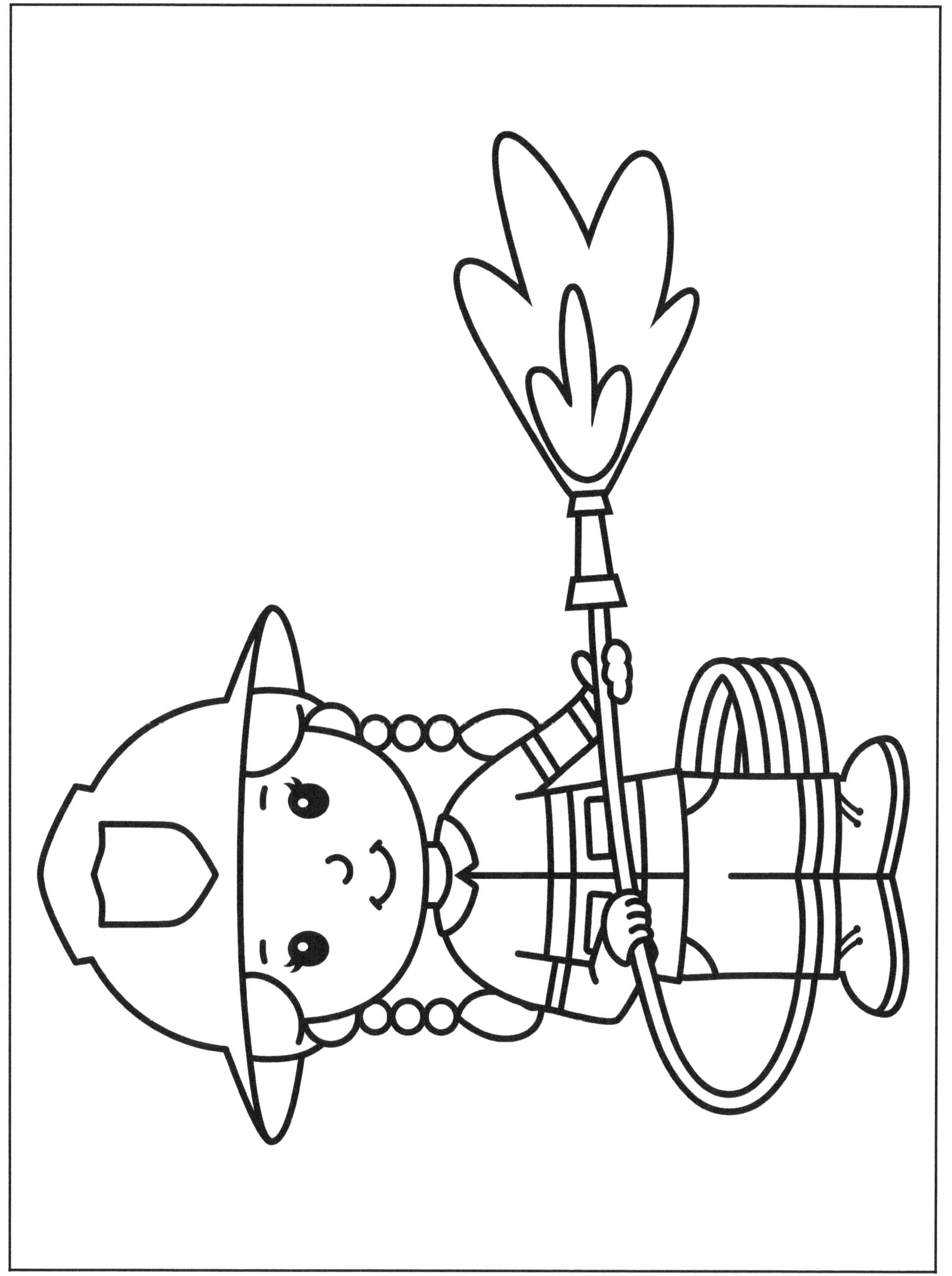

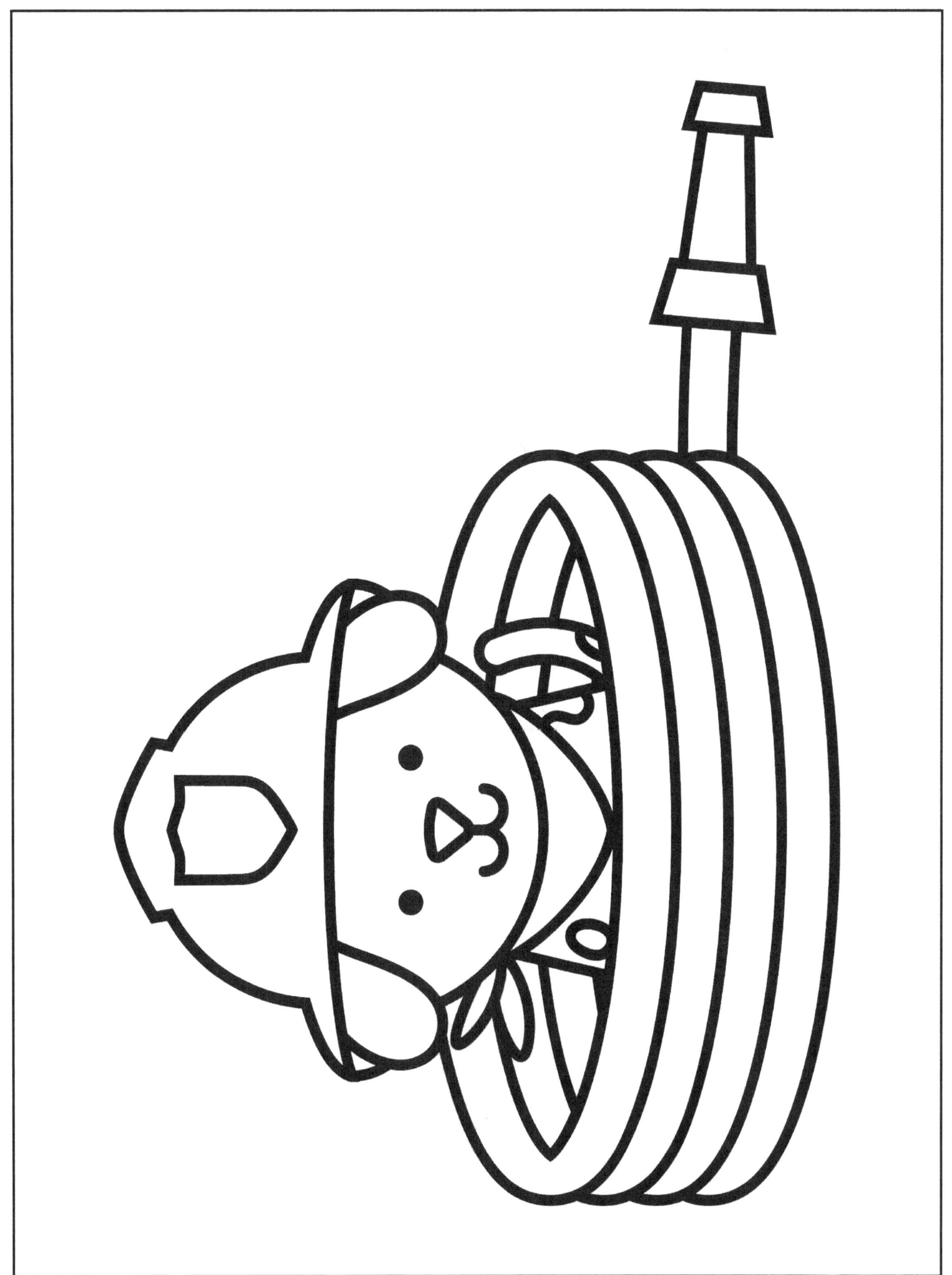

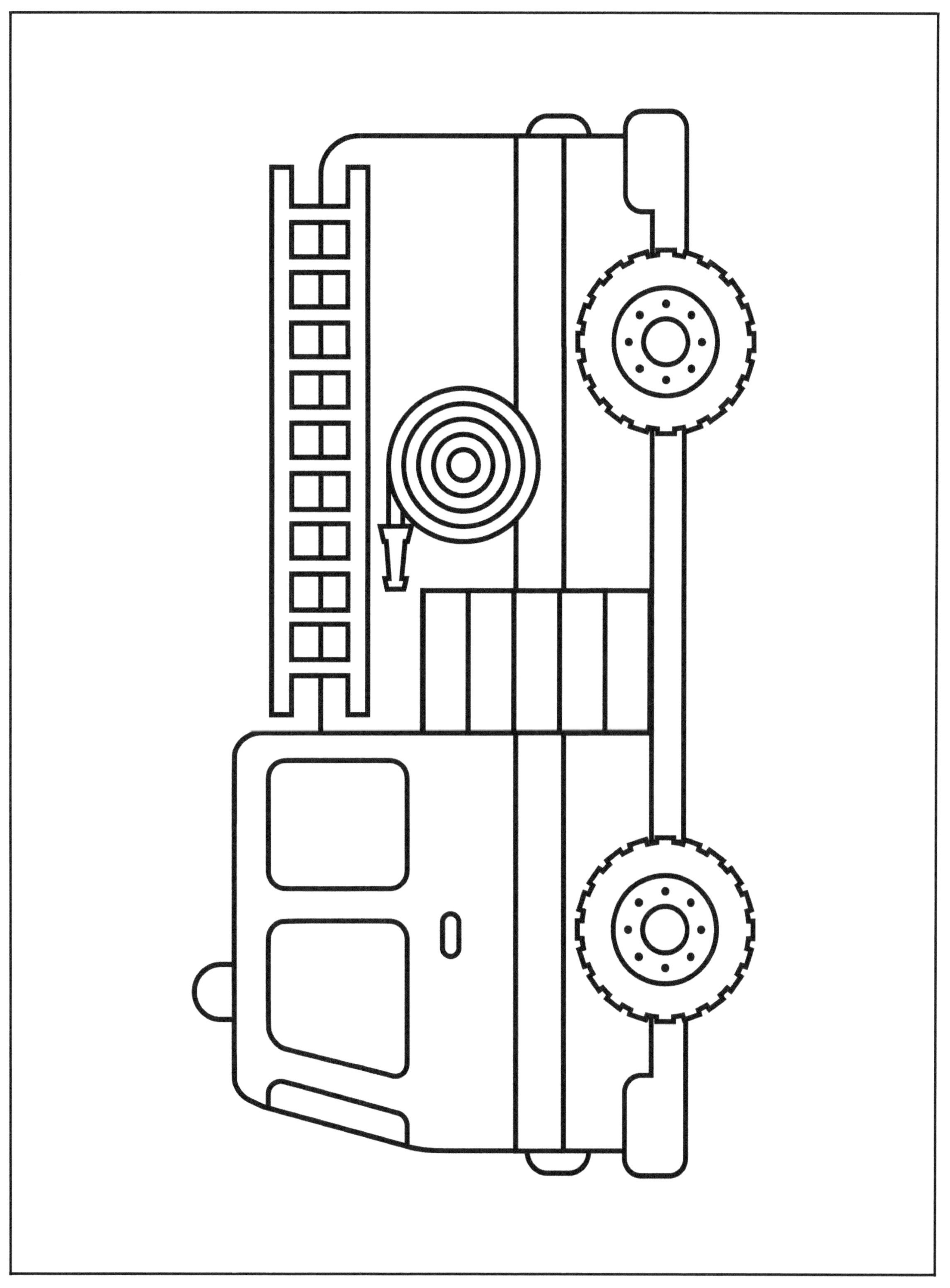

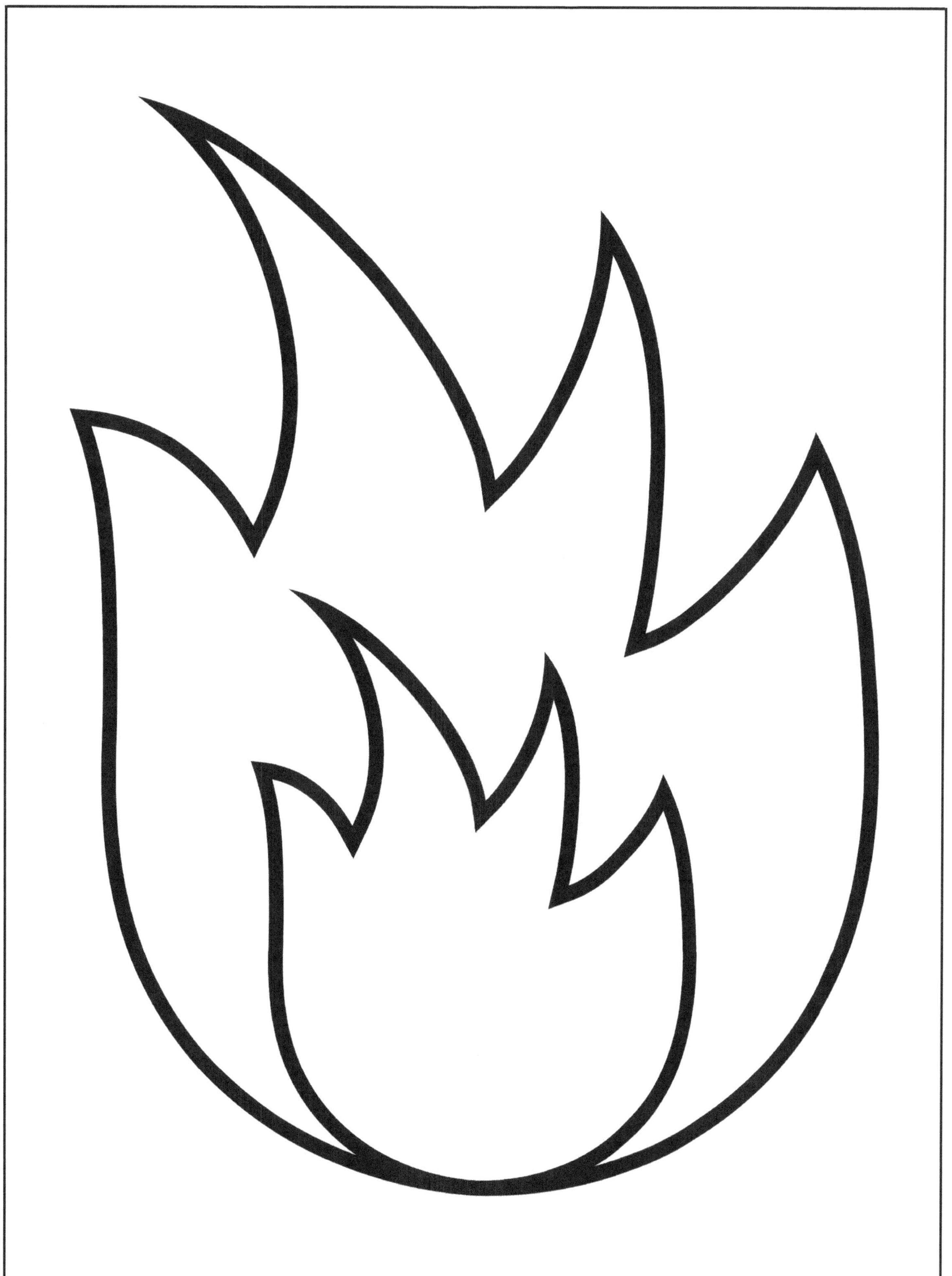

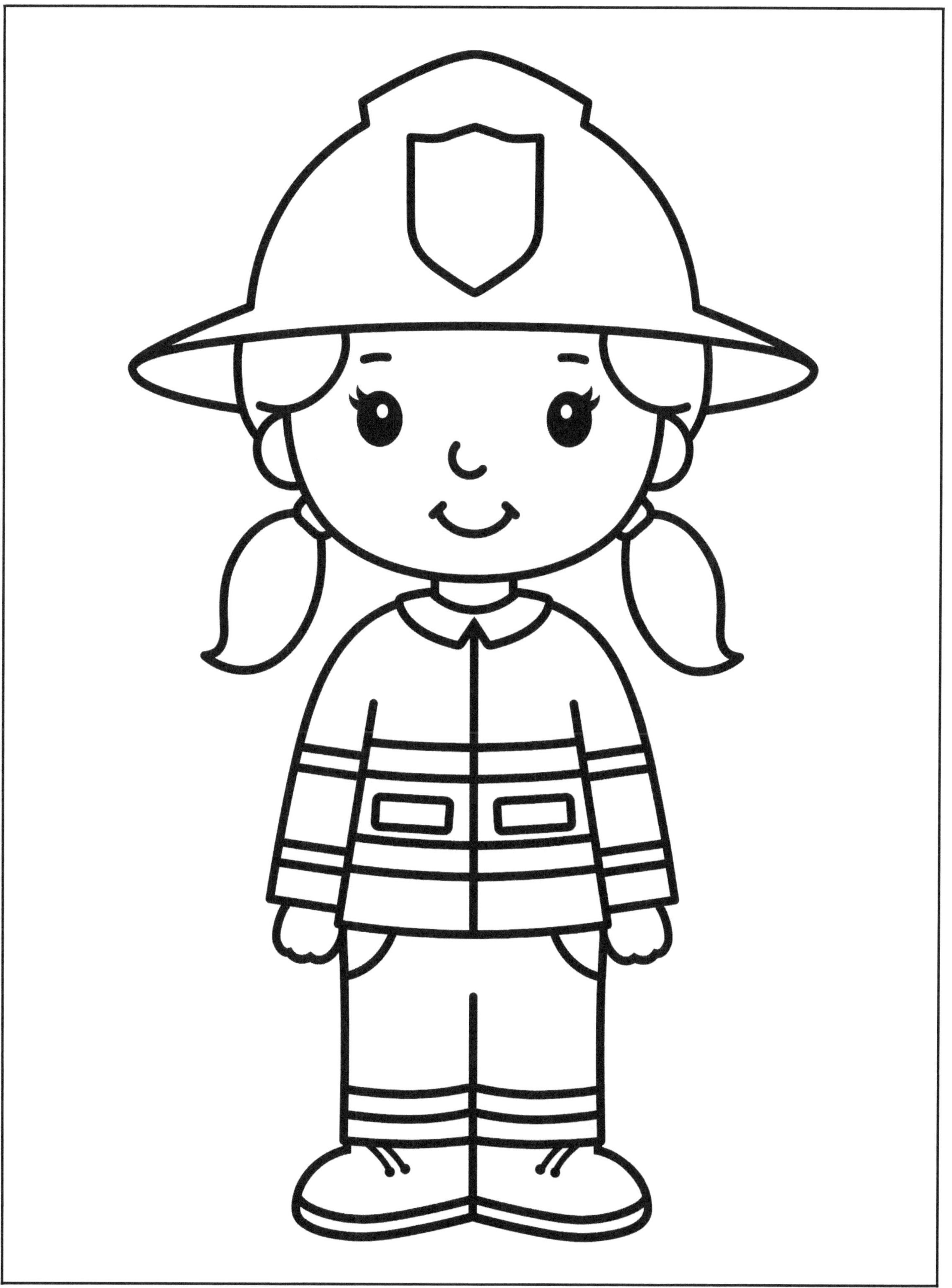

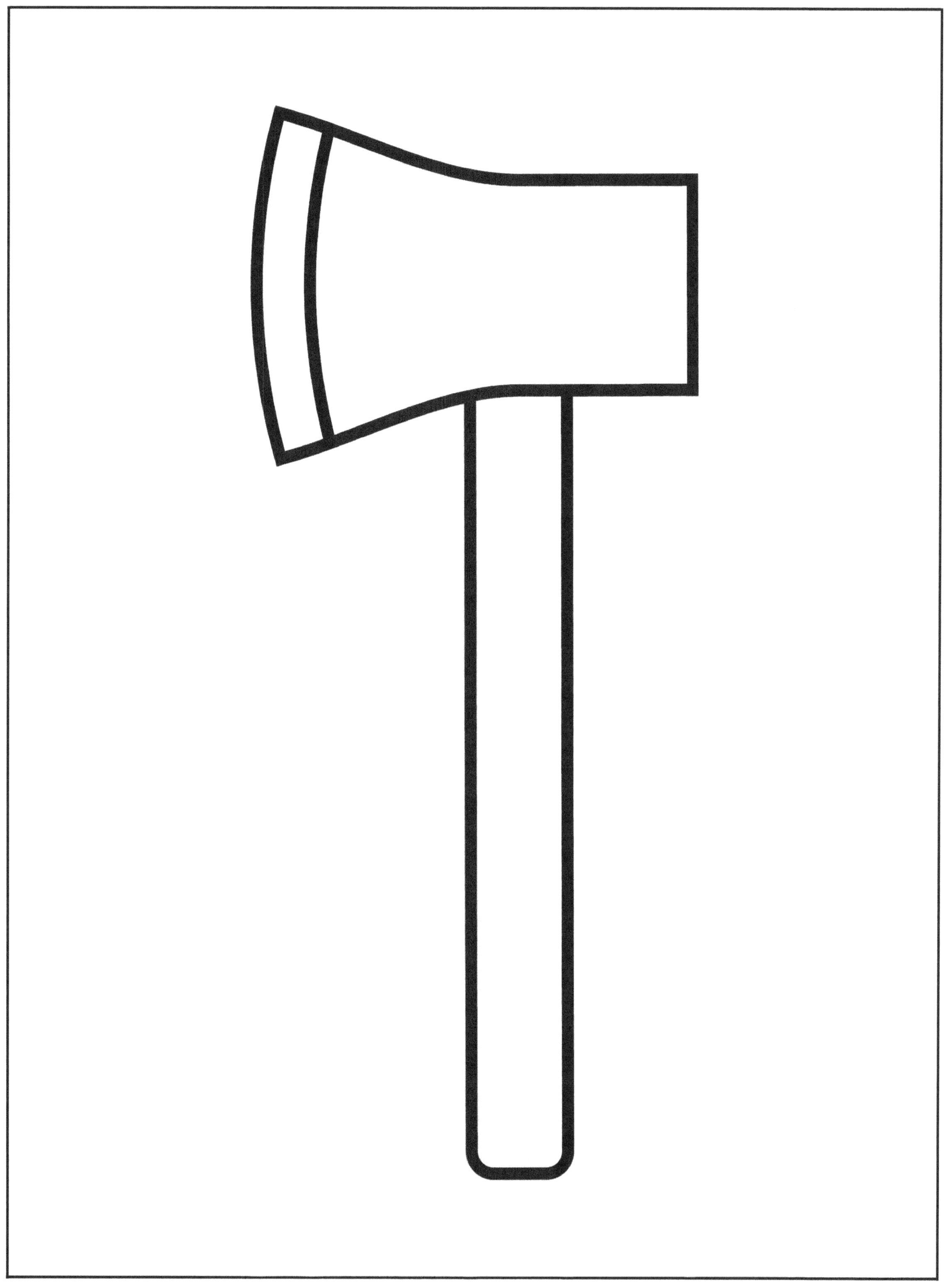

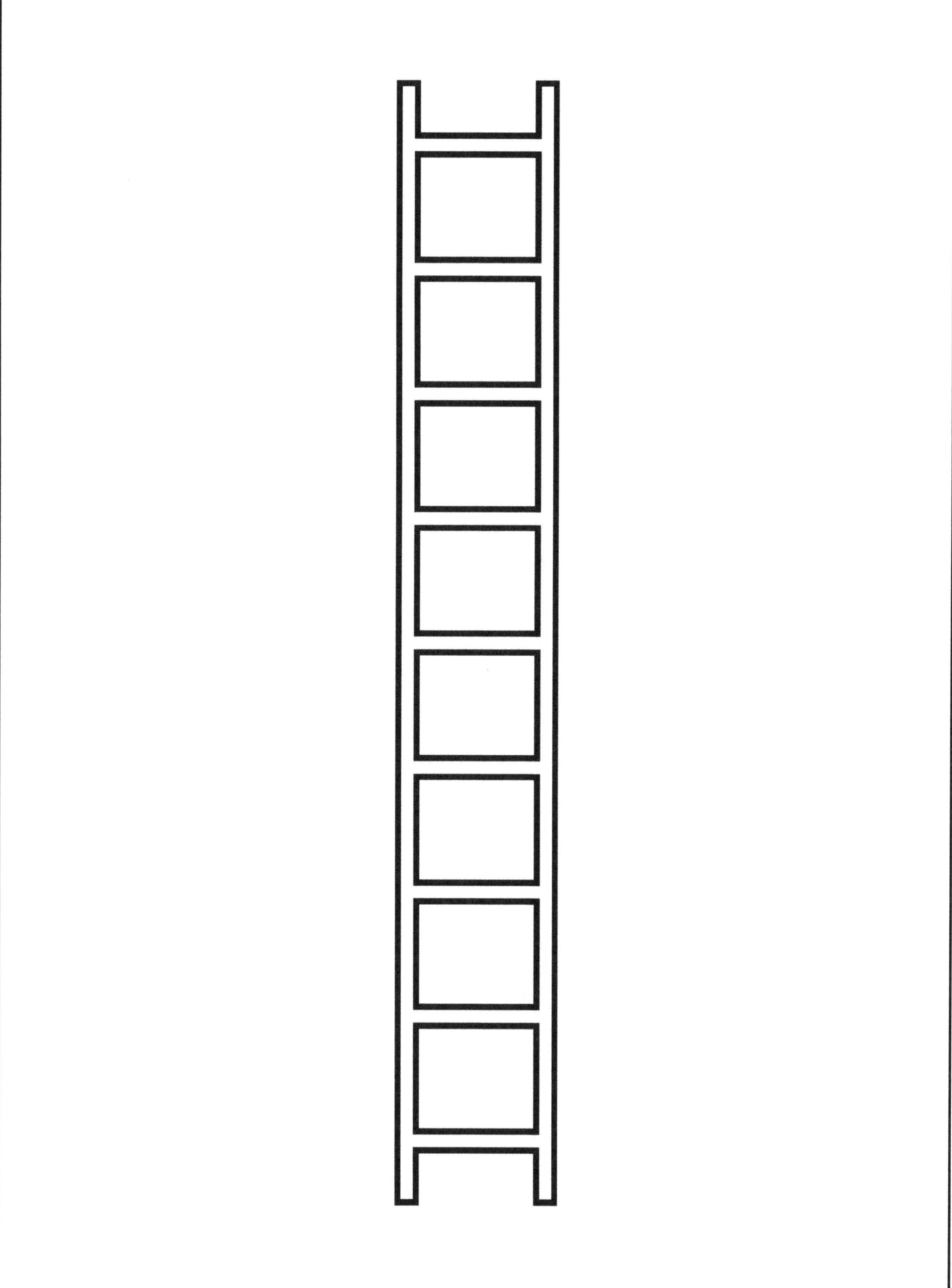

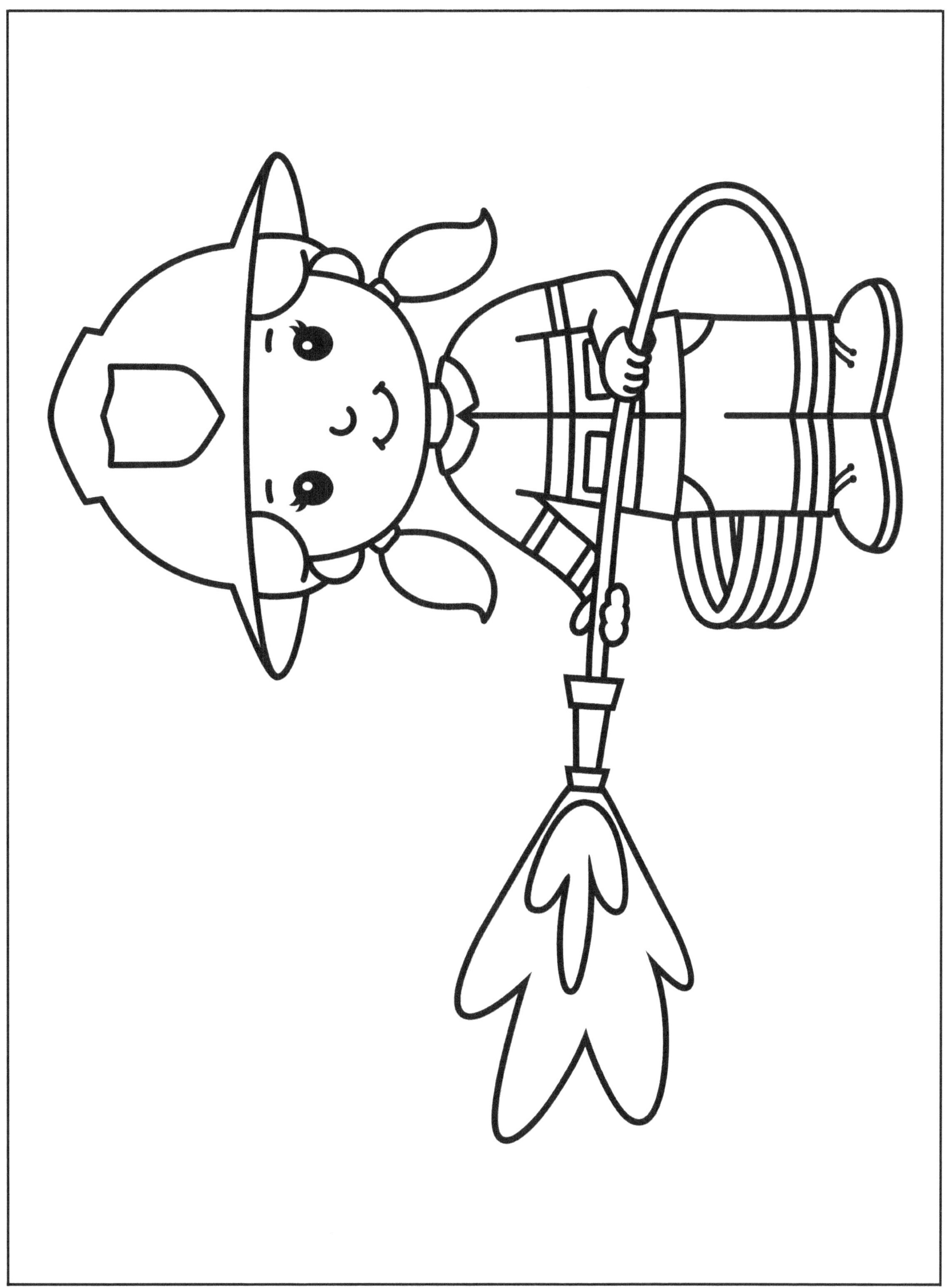

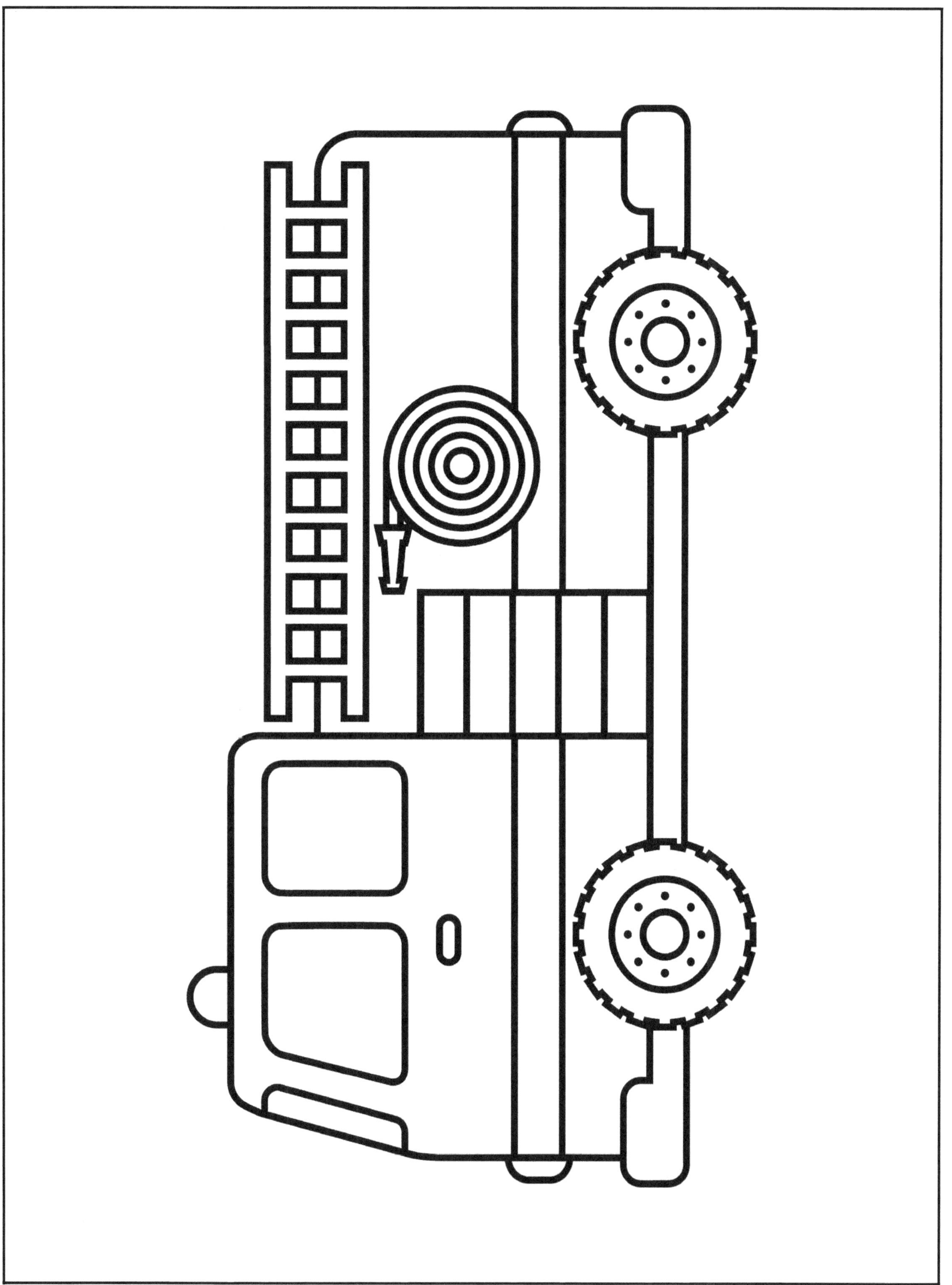

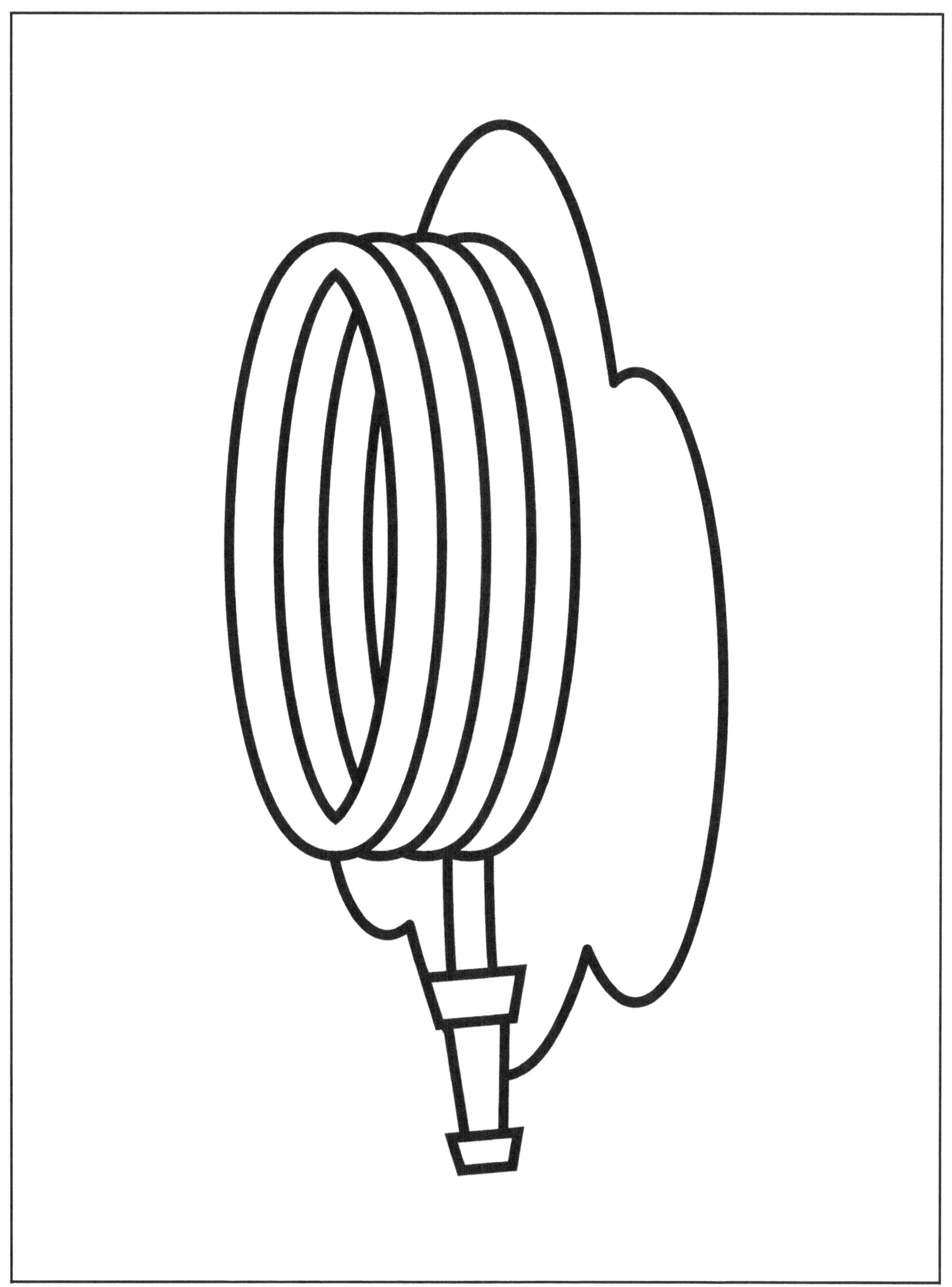

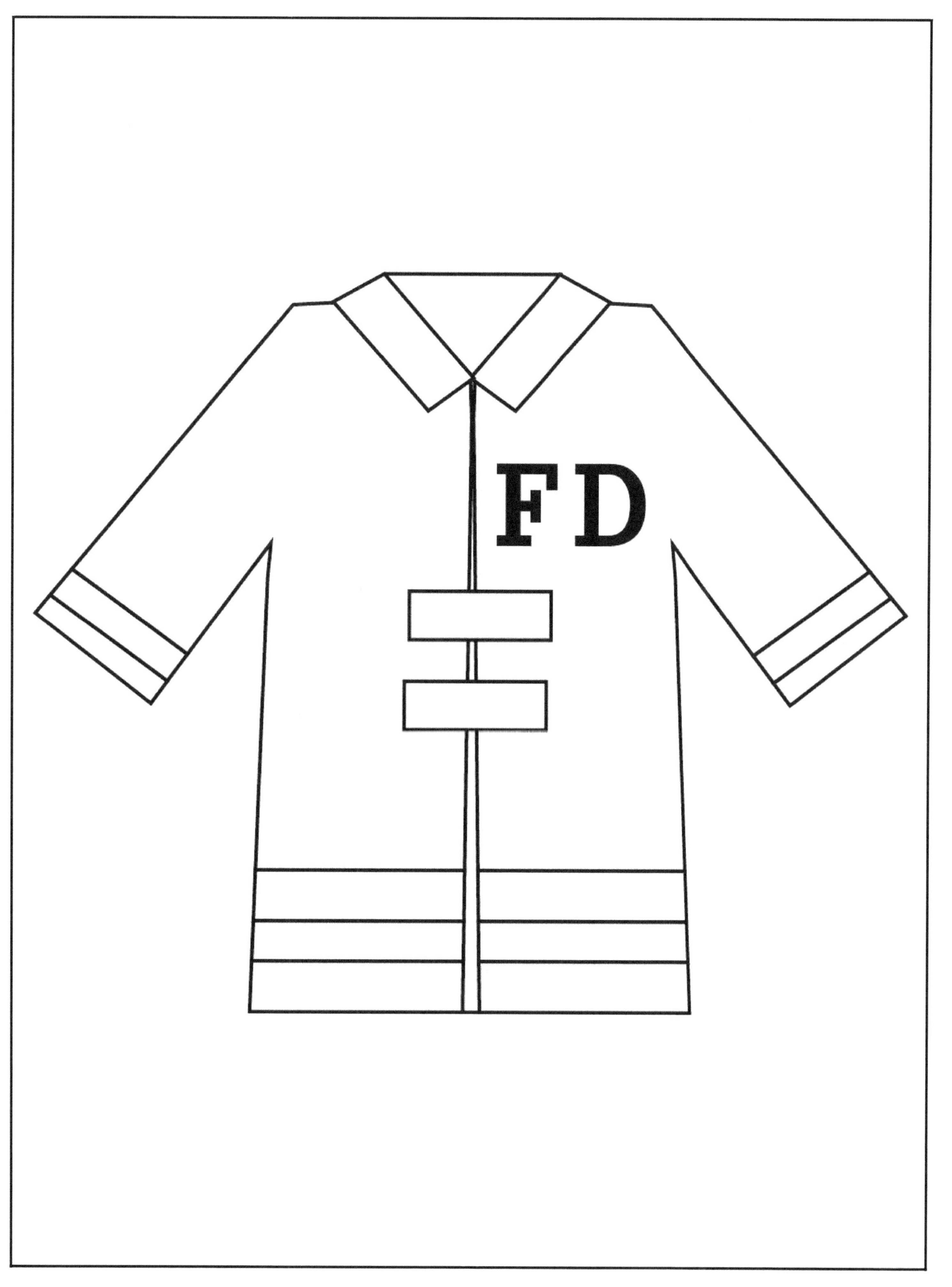

FD

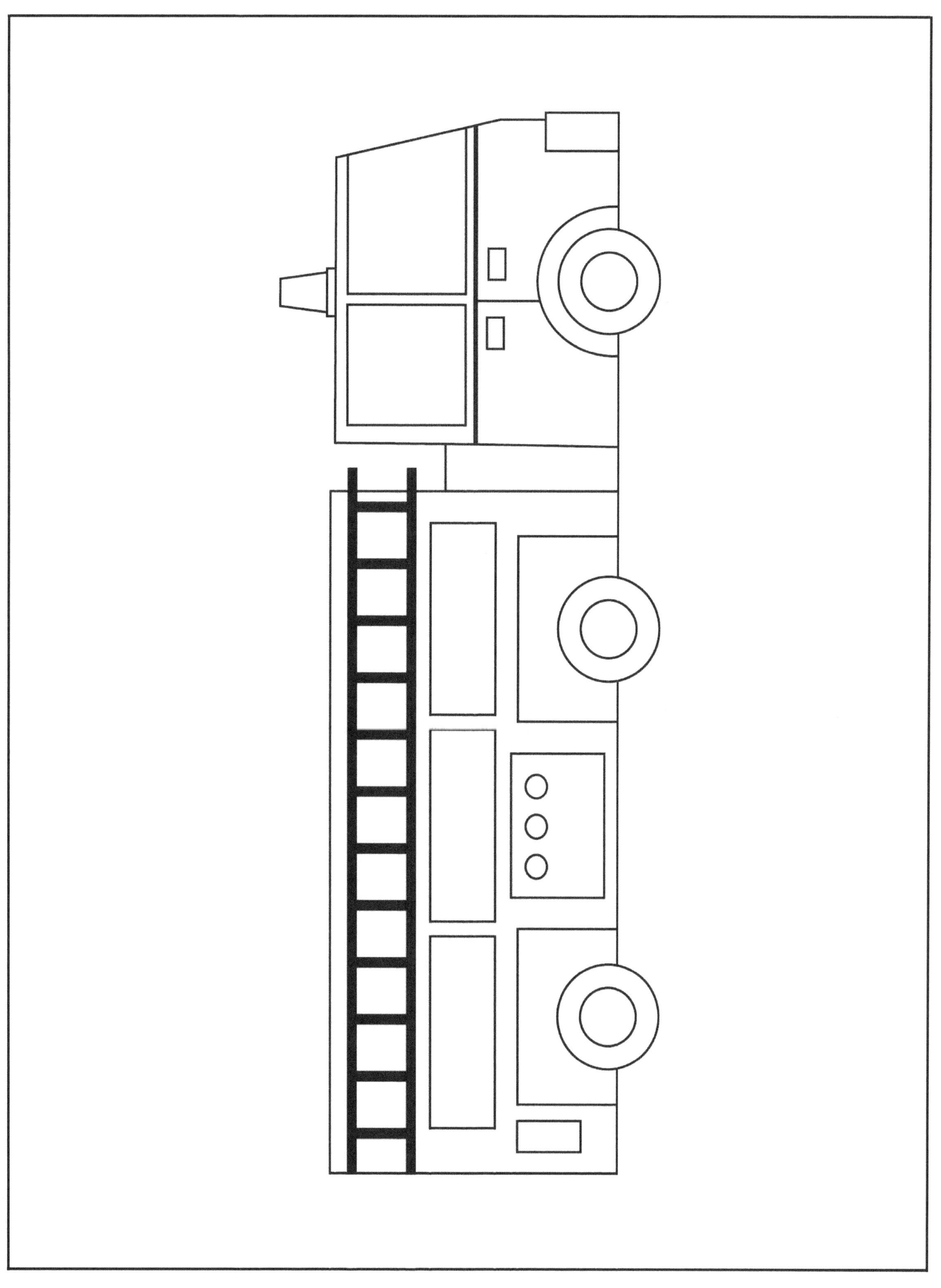

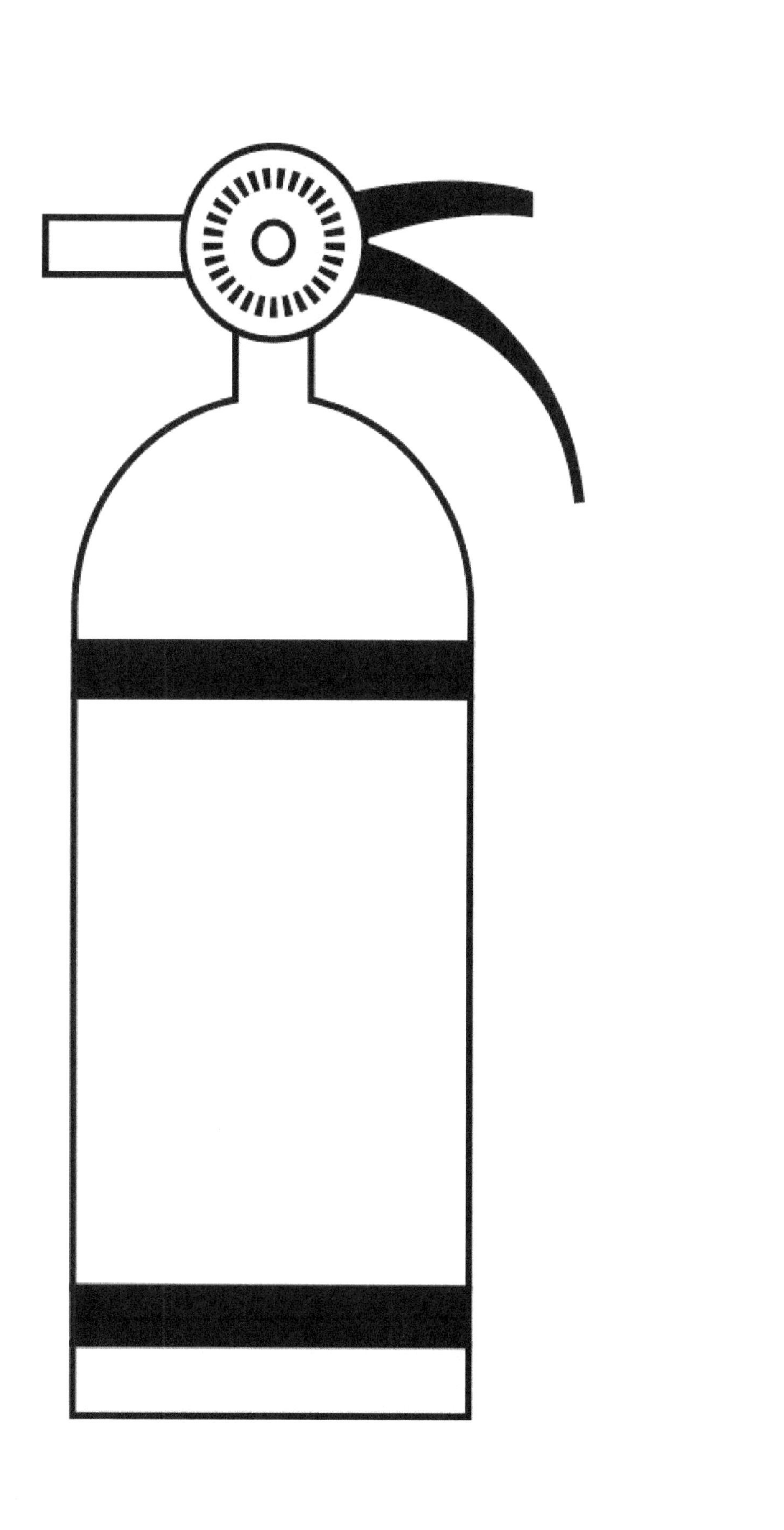

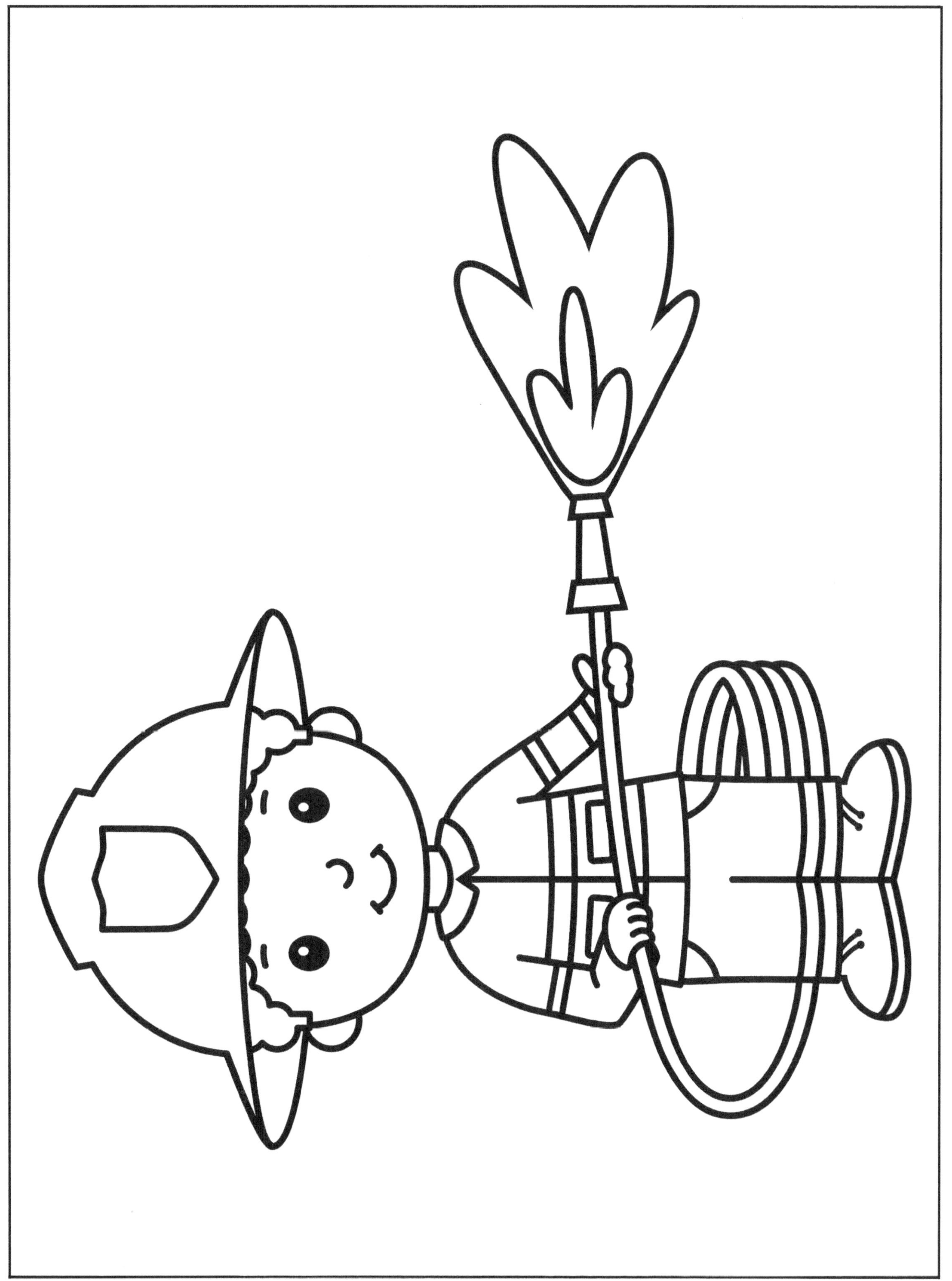

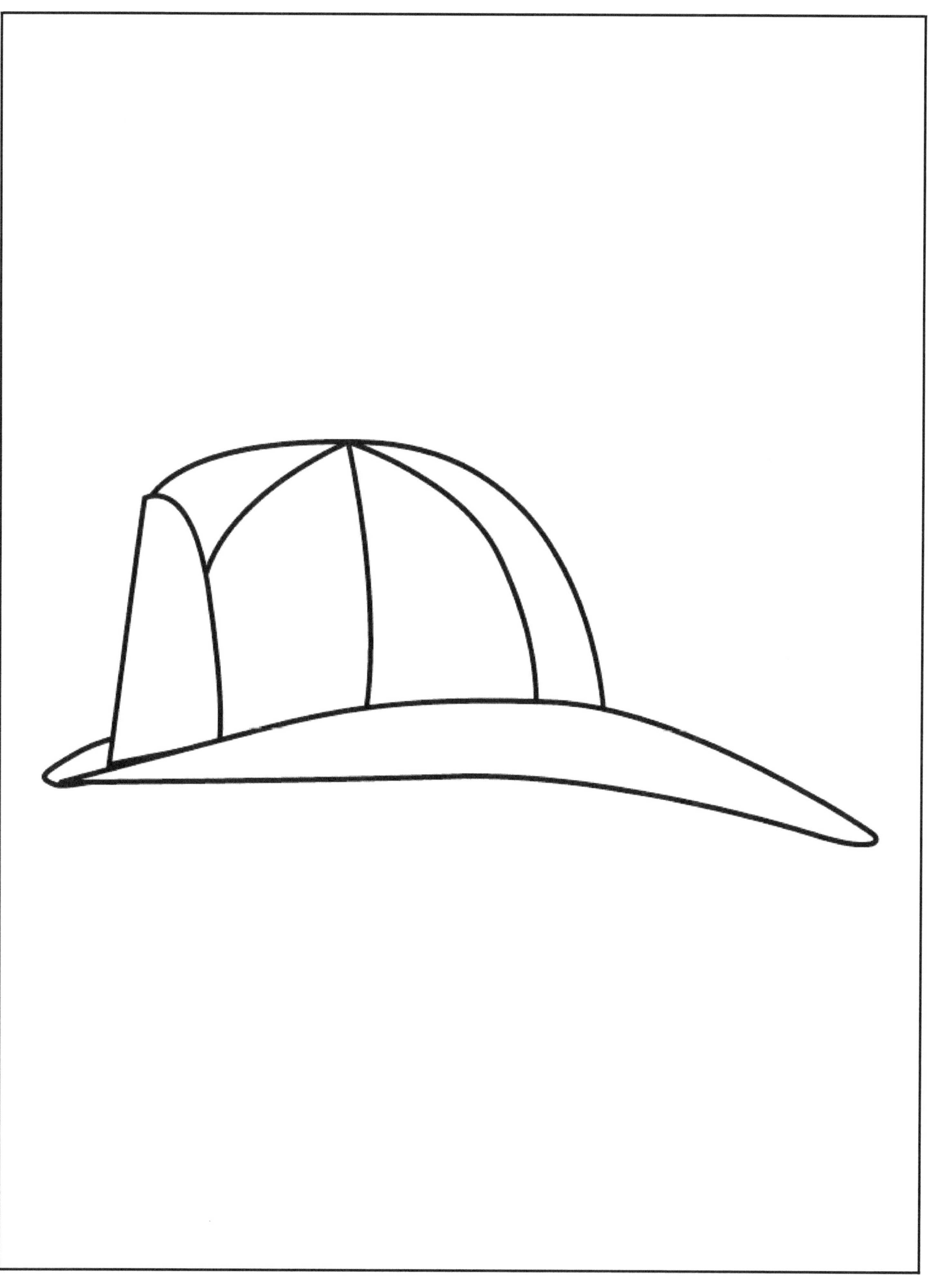

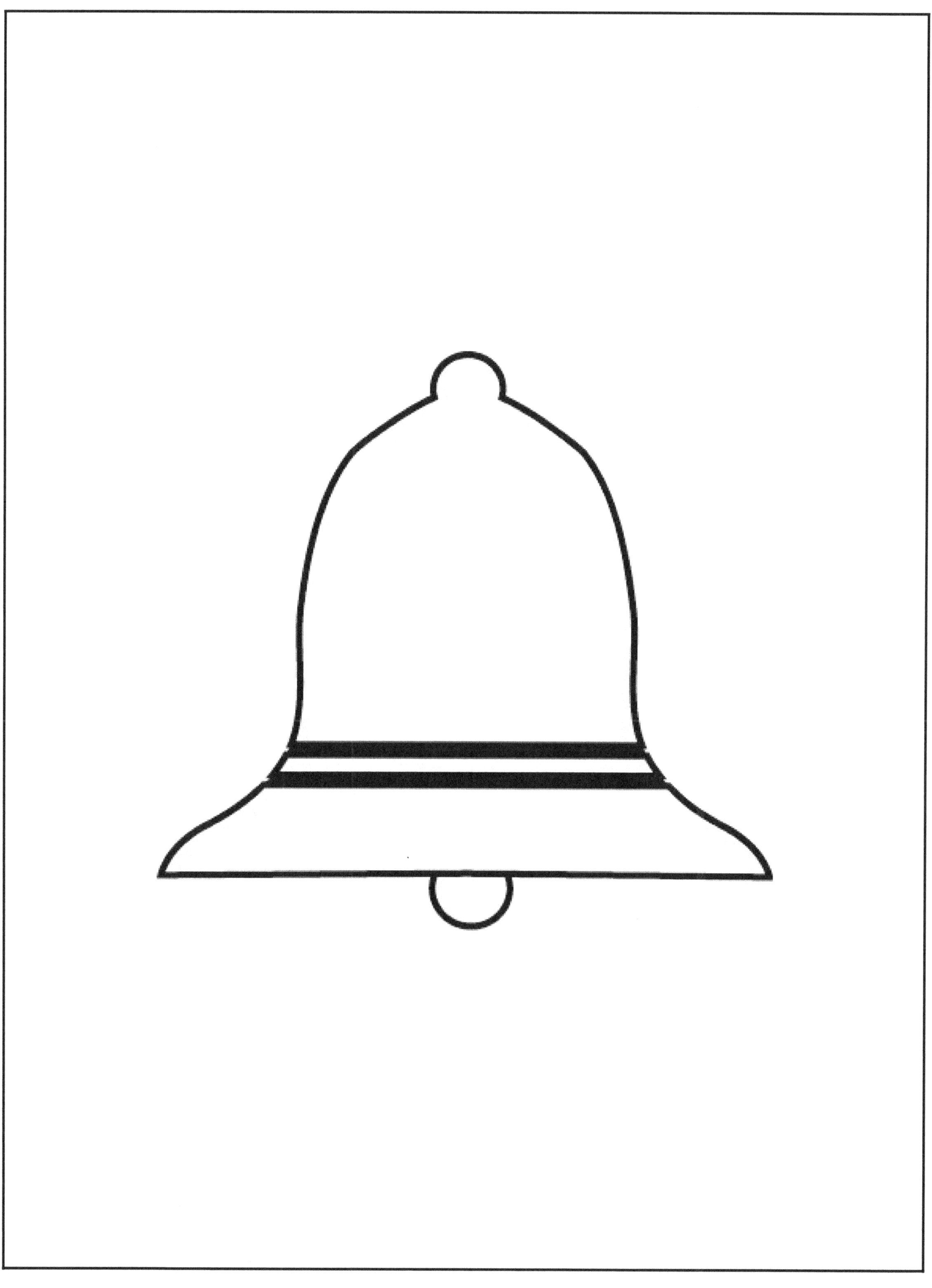

www.ingramcontent.com/pod-product-compliance
Lightning Source LLC
Chambersburg PA
CBHW081634250726
48657CB00009B/2871